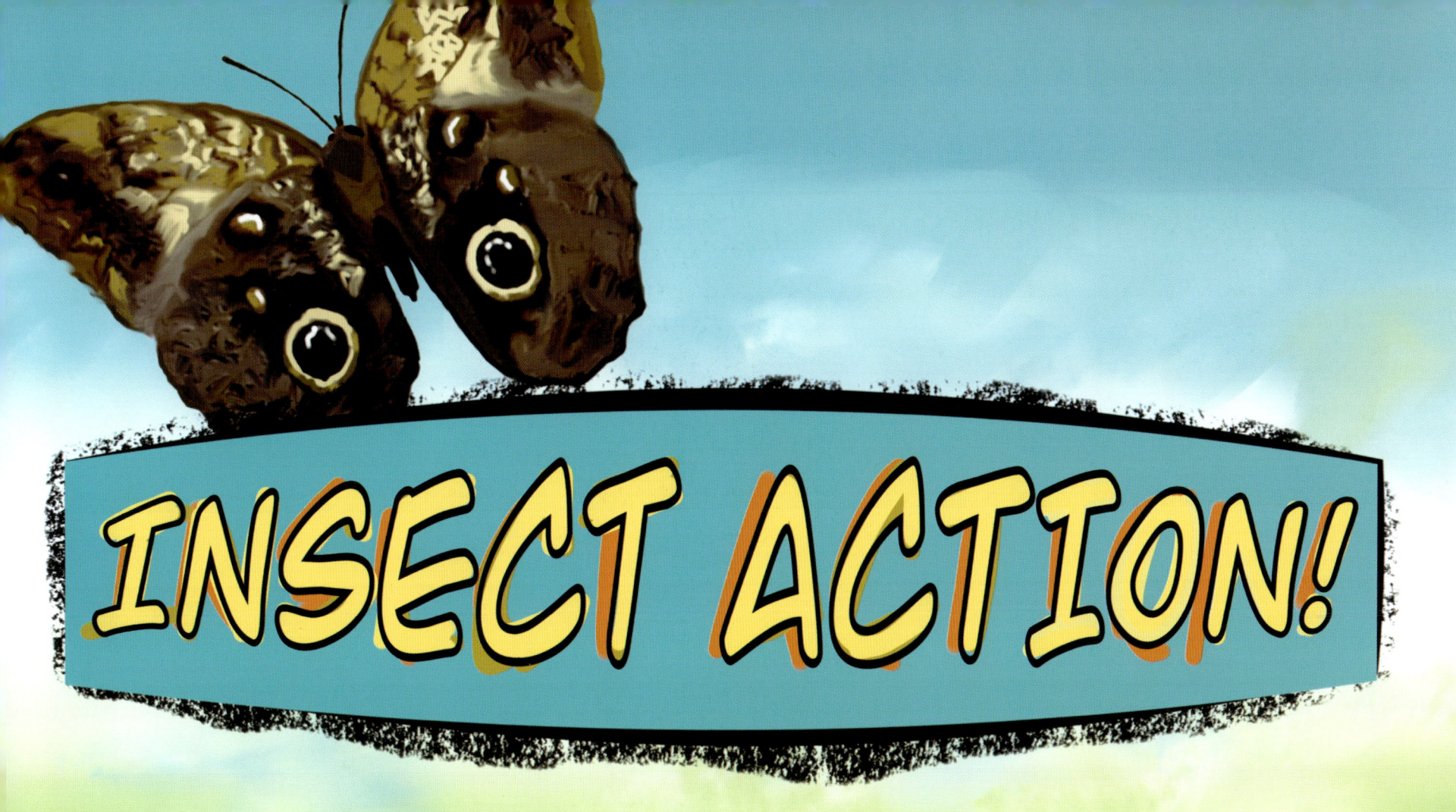

INSECT ACTION!

An Alphabet, Rhyming, and Movement Book

Written by **Heidi Braun**   Illustrated by **Sally Johnson**

Heidi Braun

This book was inspired by God's creation
and lovingly supported by my husband.

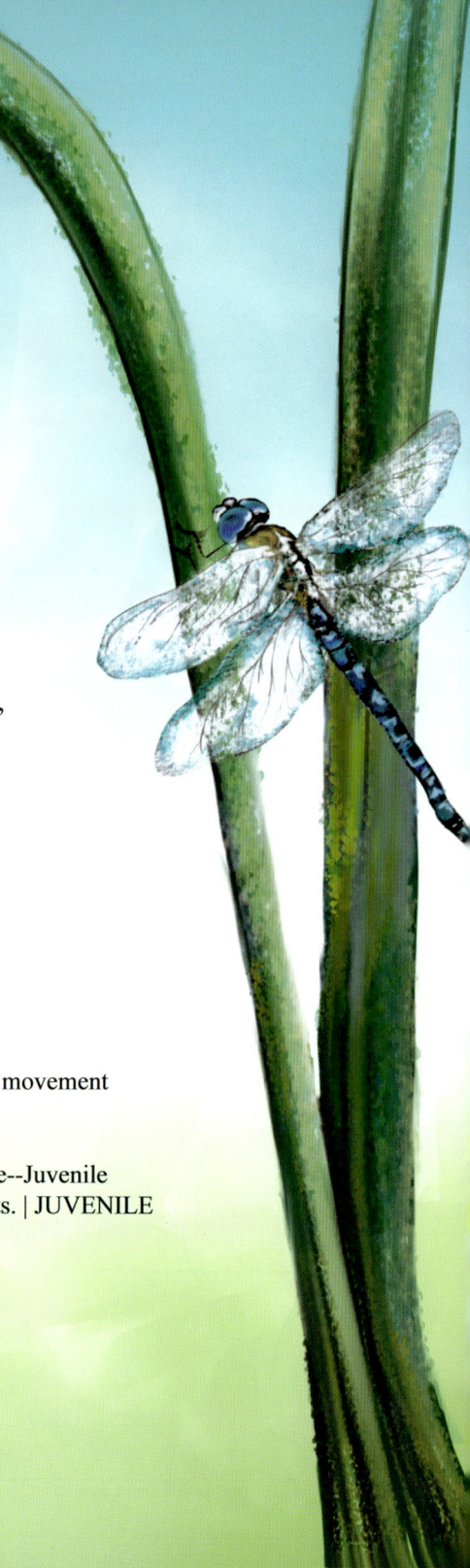

Published by Click Beetle Books LLC.
For information regarding the author and publisher, visit clickbeetlebooks.com.

Illustrated by Sally Johnson
Edited by Emily Nicholls
First edition 2024

Publisher's Cataloging-in-Publication data

Names: Braun, Heidi E., author. | Johnson, Sally Ann, illustrator.
Title: Insect action! An alphabet , rhyming , and movement book / written by Heidi Braun; illustrated by Sally Johnson.
Description: Winona, MN: Click Beetle Books LLC, 2024. | Summary: Hop like a planthopper or sway like a walking stick. Engaging movement activities, lively rhyming text, and enchanting illustrations adorn this alphabet book about insects.
Identifiers: LCCN: 2024902061 | ISBN: 979-8-9899342-0-1
Subjects: LCSH Insects--Juvenile literature. | Alphabet--Juvenile literature. | English language--Alphabet--Juvenile literature. | Exercise--Juvenile literature. | Alphabet books. | BISAC JUVENILE NONFICTION / Concepts / Alphabet | JUVENILE NONFICTION / Animals / Insects. | JUVENILE NONFICTION / Health & Daily Living / Fitness & Exercise
Classification: LCC QL467.2 .B73 2024 | DDC 595.7--dc23

Printed in the USA

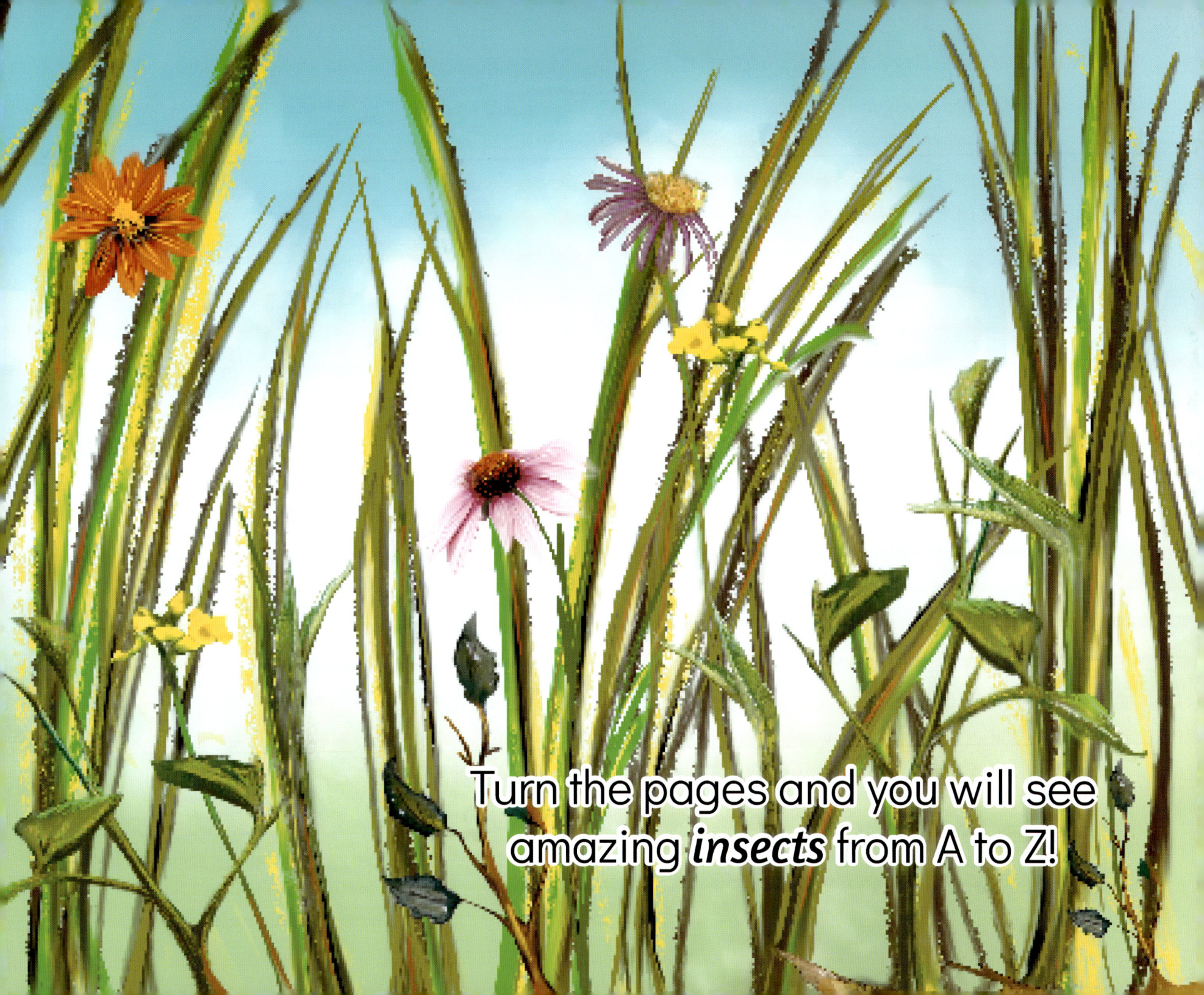

Turn the pages and you will see amazing *insects* from A to Z!

Aa

acrobat ant

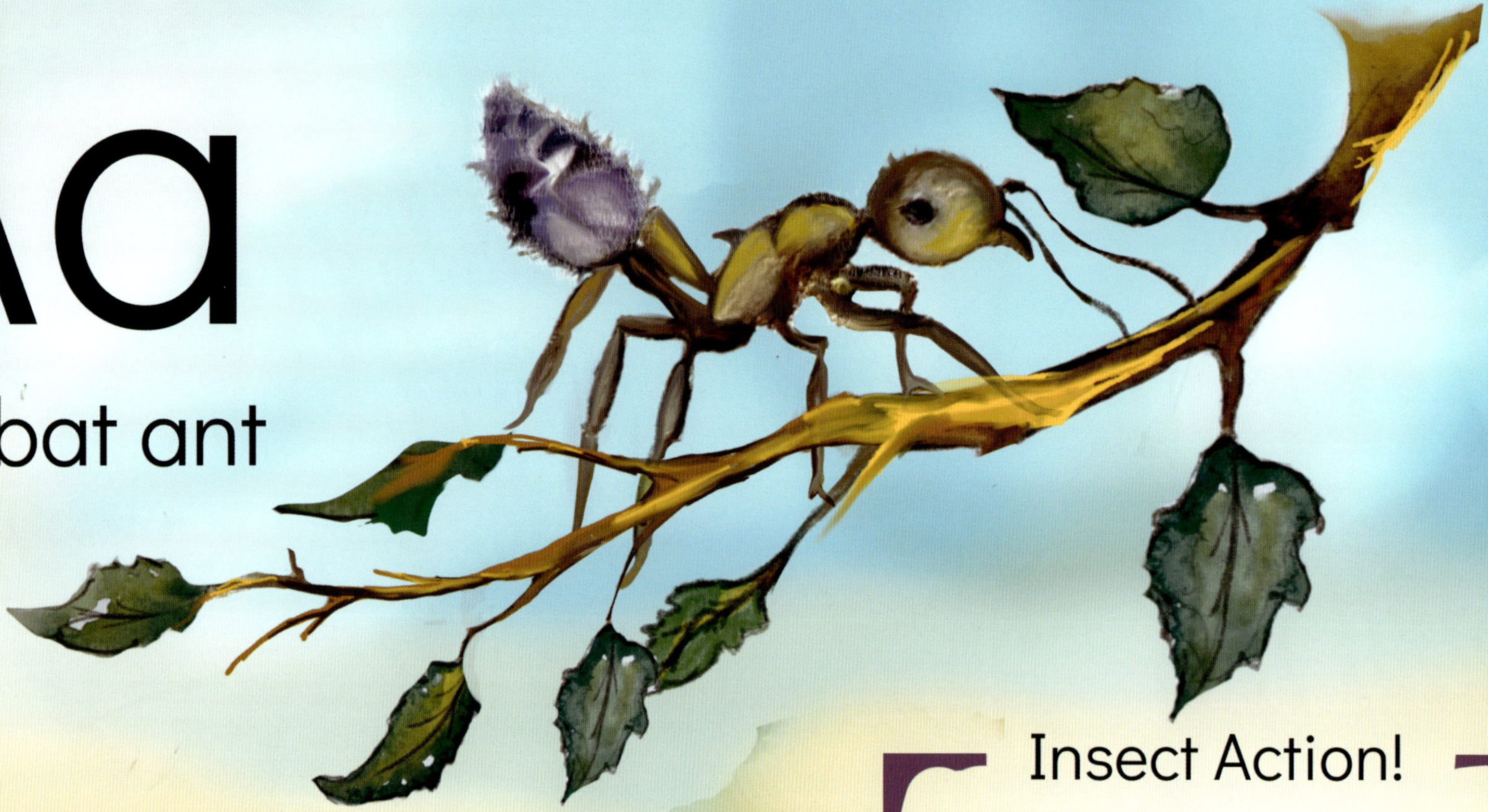

Acrobat ant lifts its **abdomen** high, raising it up toward the sky.

When acrobat ants become frightened, they raise their abdomens.

Insect Action!

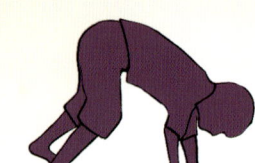

Walk with your hands on the floor and your bottom up like an acrobat ant.

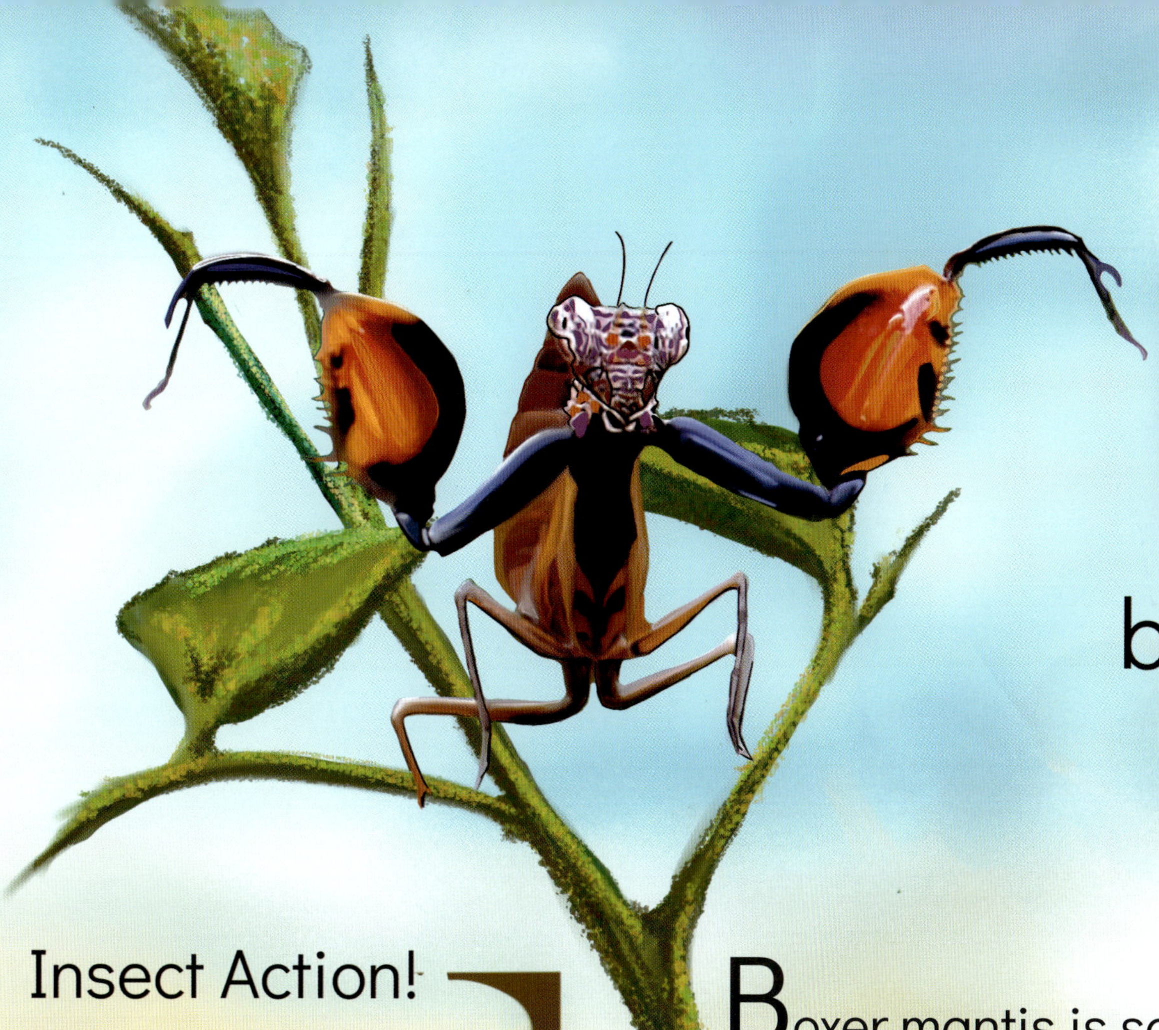

Bb

boxer mantis

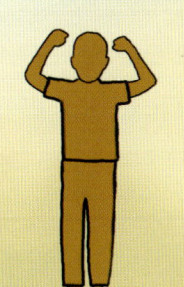

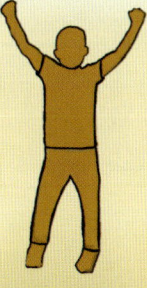

Boxer mantis is so strong;
it grabs with forelegs stretched out long.

Boxer mantises have long, strong front legs, or forelegs, which they use like arms. They use these special legs to reach, grab, and ***communicate*** with other mantises.

Insect Action!

Bend your arms and then stretch them high like a boxer mantis.

Cc

click beetle

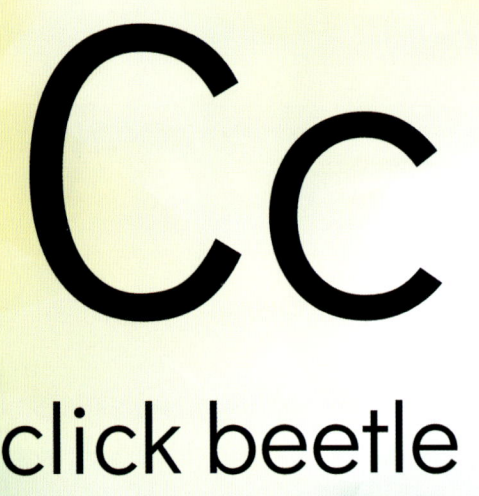

Click beetle falls flat on its back.
With one quick flip, it's back on track.

Click beetles make a clicking sound when
they flip from their backs onto their feet.

Insect Action!

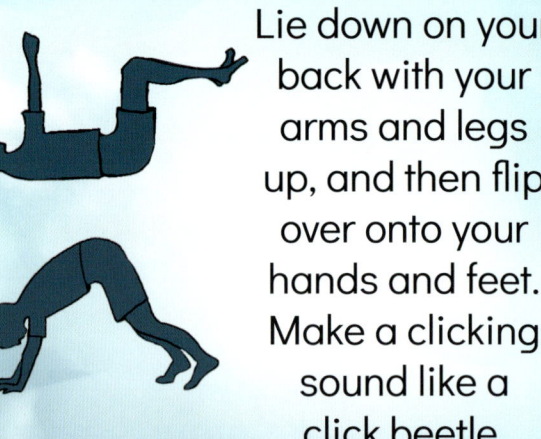

Lie down on your back with your arms and legs up, and then flip over onto your hands and feet. Make a clicking sound like a click beetle.

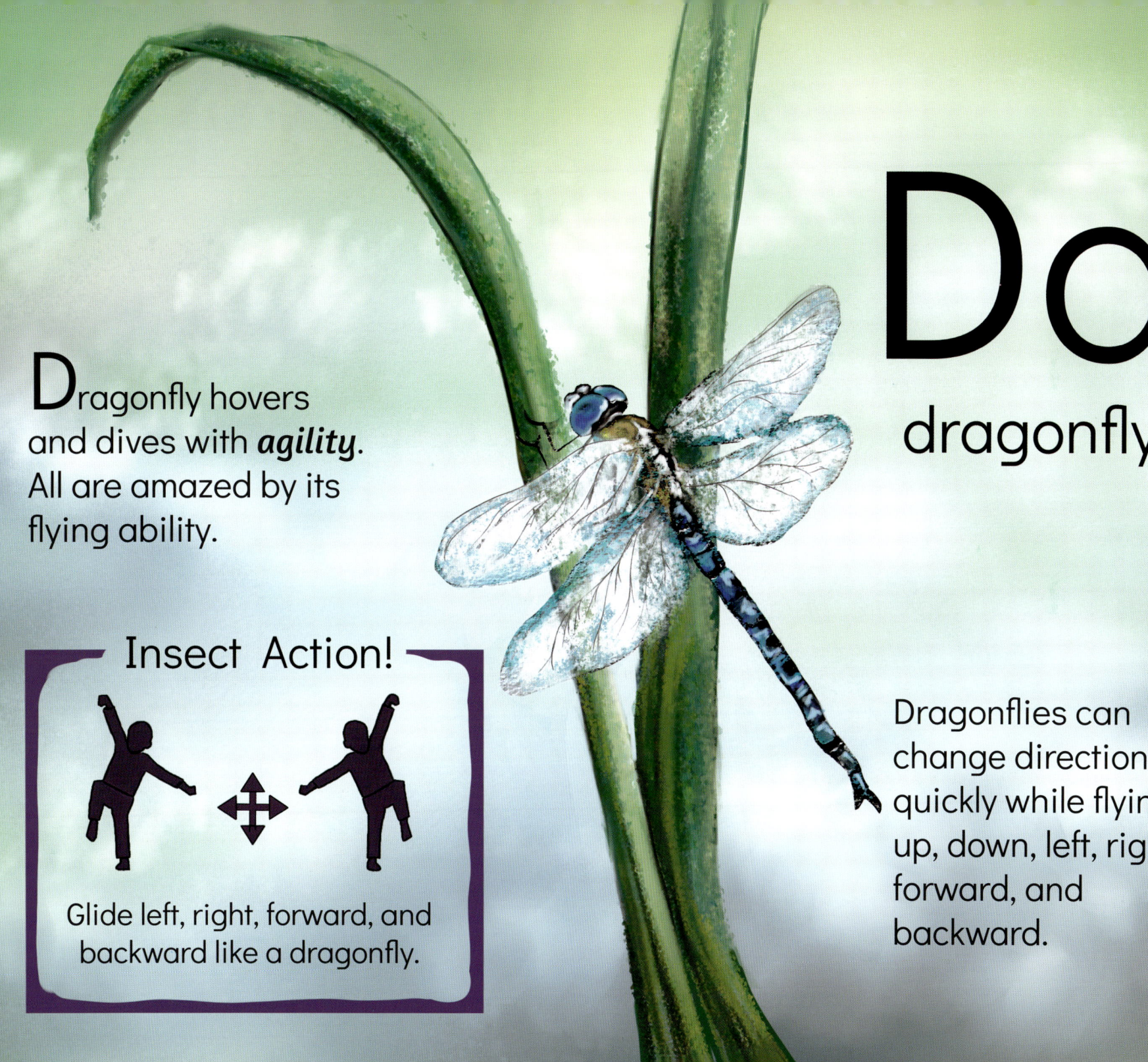

Dd
dragonfly

Dragonfly hovers and dives with *agility*. All are amazed by its flying ability.

Insect Action!

Glide left, right, forward, and backward like a dragonfly.

Dragonflies can change direction quickly while flying: up, down, left, right, forward, and backward.

Ee

elephant hawk moth

Elephant hawk moth hovers at night, feeding on flowers 'til dawn's early light.

Elephant hawk moths hover while sipping nectar from flowers. They are **nocturnal** insects.

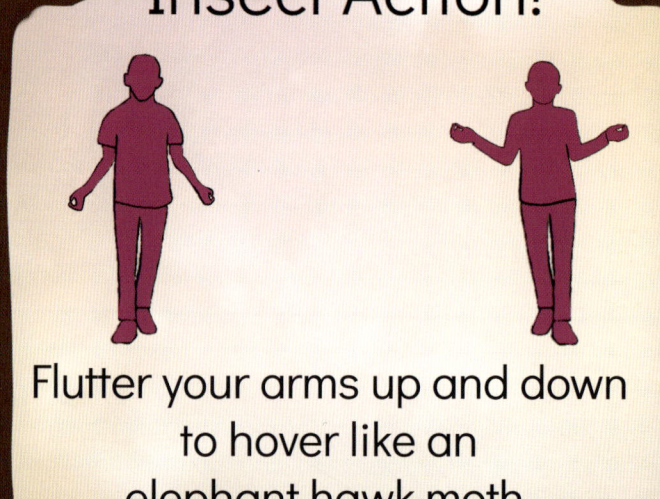

Insect Action!

Flutter your arms up and down to hover like an elephant hawk moth.

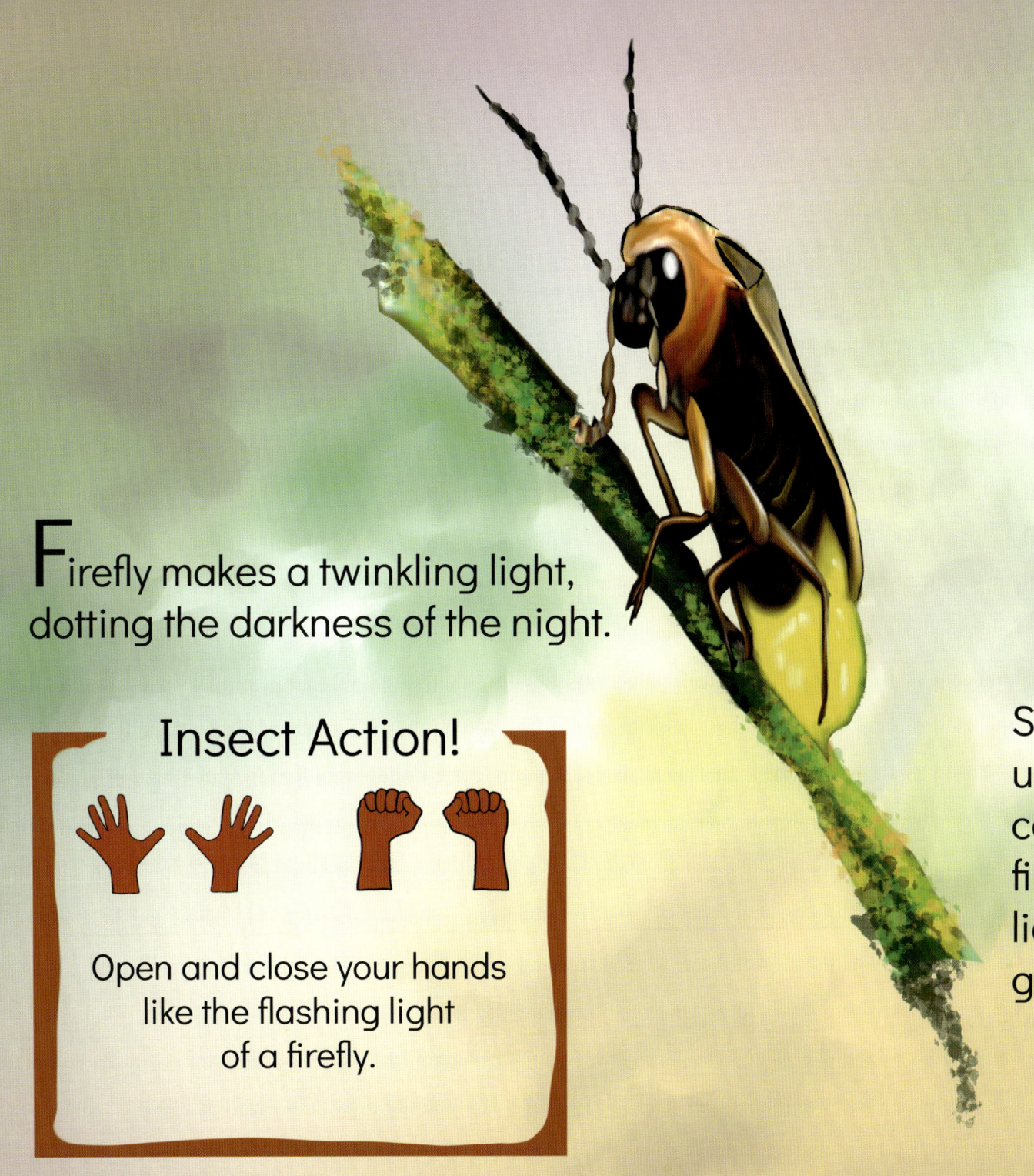

Ff
firefly

Firefly makes a twinkling light,
dotting the darkness of the night.

Some fireflies light
up their abdomens to
communicate or to
find a mate. Firefly
light can be yellow,
green, or orange.

Insect Action!

Open and close your hands
like the flashing light
of a firefly.

Gg

grasshopper

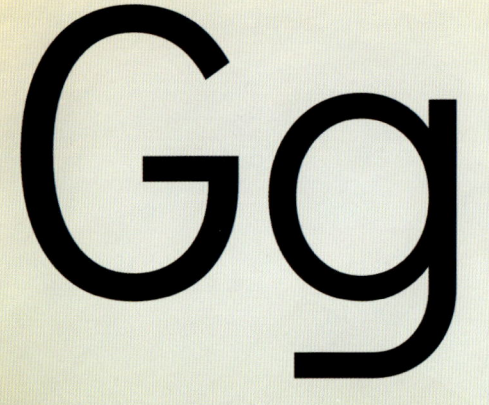

Grasshopper quickly hops on by,
strong legs **propelling** it very high.

Grasshoppers are good fliers and jumpers.
They can jump many times their body
length.

Insect Action!

Bend your knees, and then
jump up high like a
grasshopper.

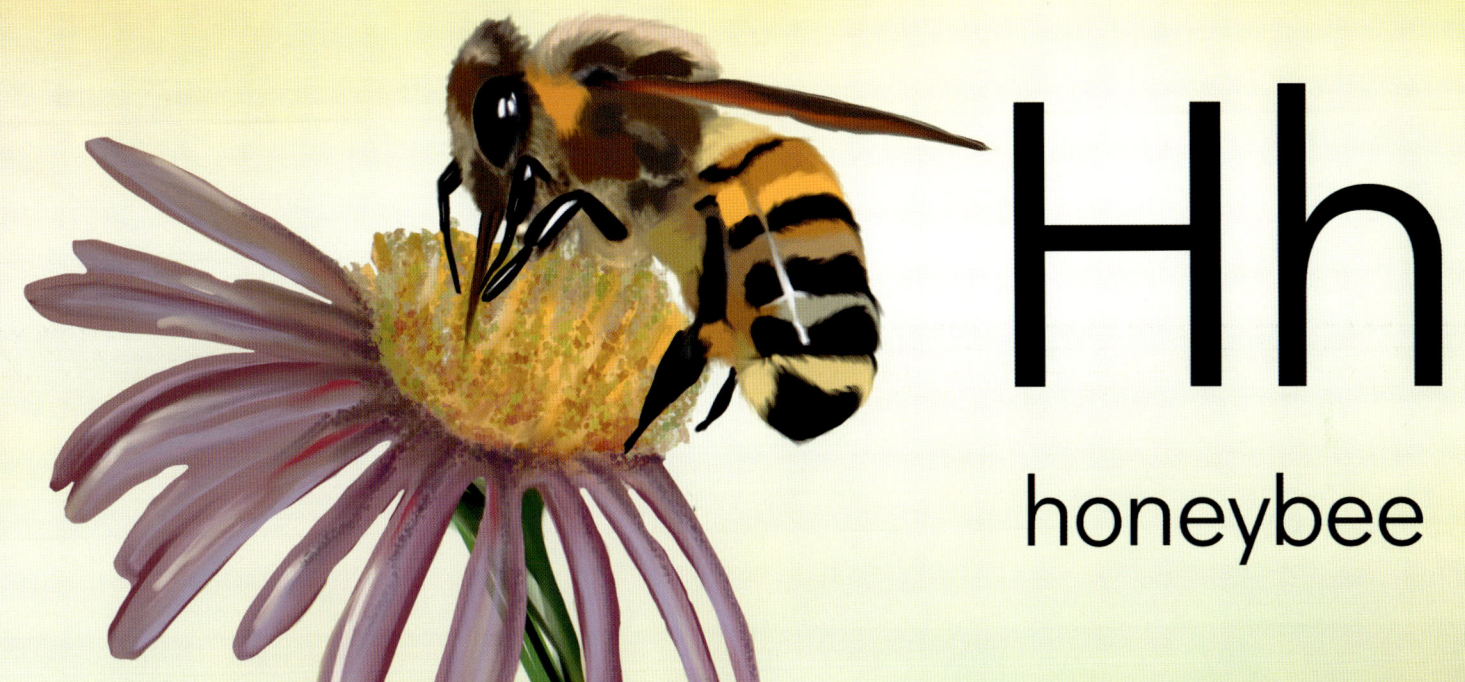

Hh
honeybee

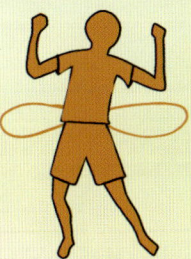
Honeybee dances in a figure-eight, telling others where food is great.

Honeybees tell other honeybees where to find food by dancing in a circle or a figure-eight, depending on where the food is located.

I i

inchworm

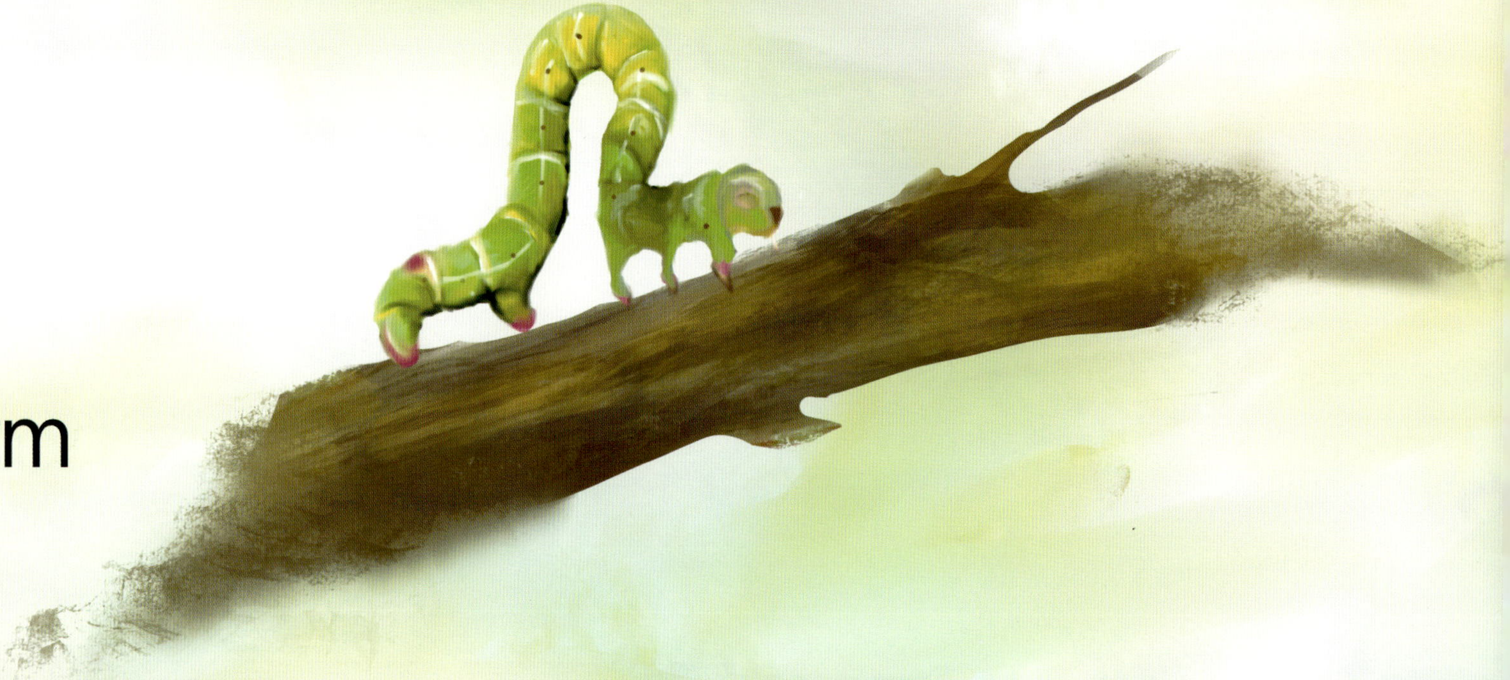

Inchworm must be very strong
to arch its back and stretch out long.

Inchworms are hairless caterpillars. They
only have legs at the ends of their bodies,
so they grab with their front legs and
bring up their rear with their back legs.

Insect Action!

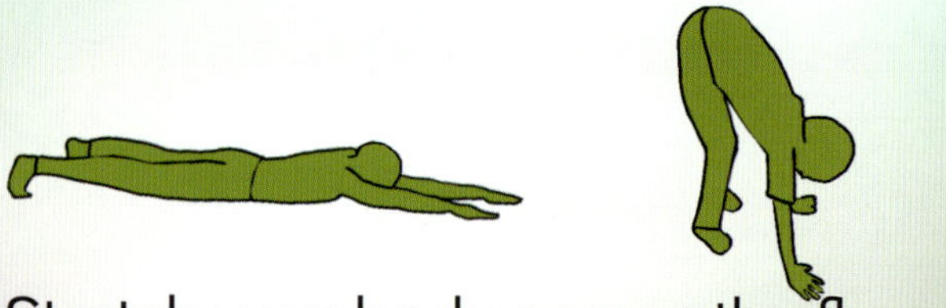

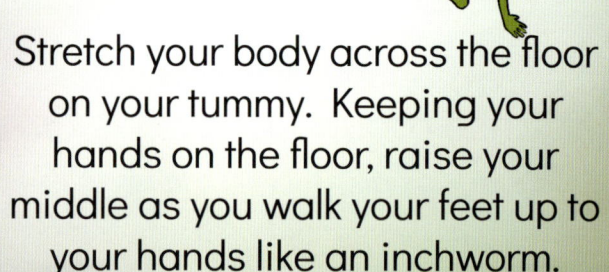

Stretch your body across the floor
on your tummy. Keeping your
hands on the floor, raise your
middle as you walk your feet up to
your hands like an inchworm.

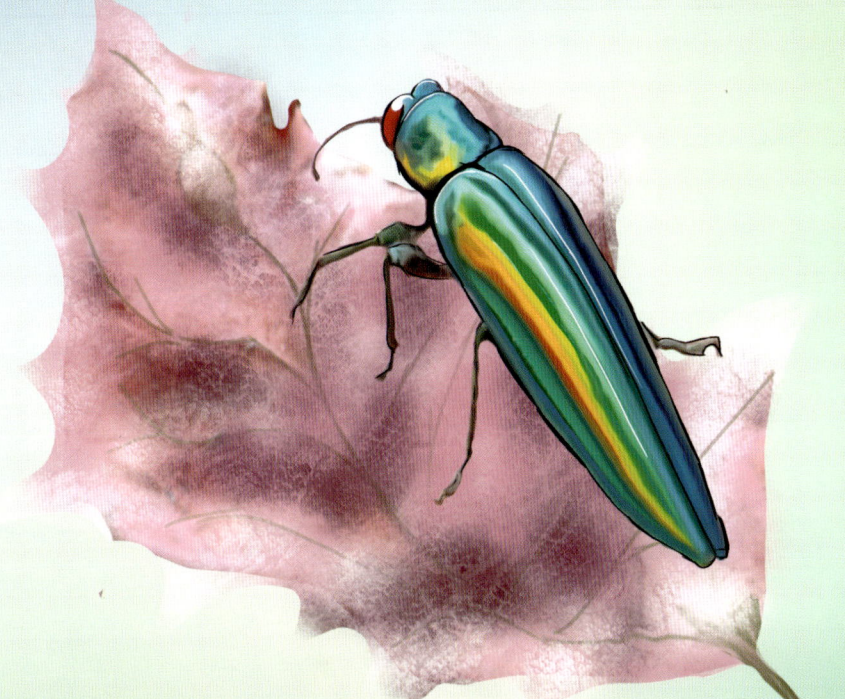

Jj

jewel beetle

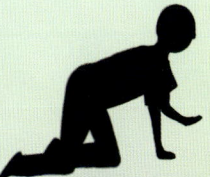
Jewel beetle scurries in almost a run. Its *iridescent* shell glimmers in the sun.

Jewel beetles are sometimes collected because of their beautiful red, blue, green, and purple colors.

Kk

katydid

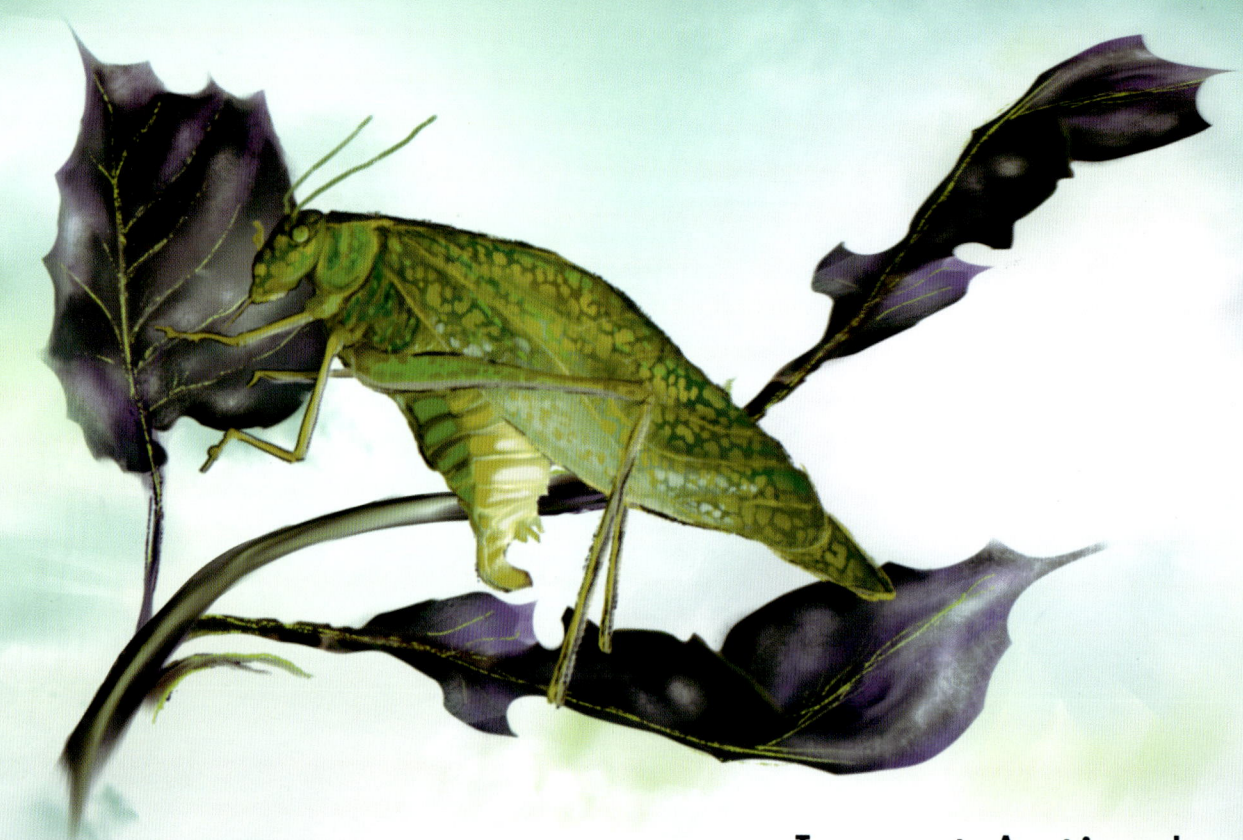

Katydid may look a bit like a cricket, tricky to find when hiding in the thicket.

Katydids are good at hiding from *predators* in leaves and grasses by using *camouflage*. They flutter their wings and leap to travel.

Insect Action!

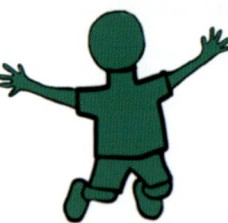

Flutter your arms up and down and leap like a katydid.

Ll

lanternfly

Lanternfly, with its silly-looking snout, ambles side to side to move about.

Insect Action!

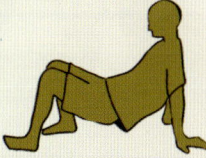

Sit with your hands on the floor behind you. Raise your bottom. Use your hands and feet to move sideways like a lanternfly.

Lanternflies use their snouts to suck sap from trees. They move sideways, walking like crabs.

Mm

mosquito

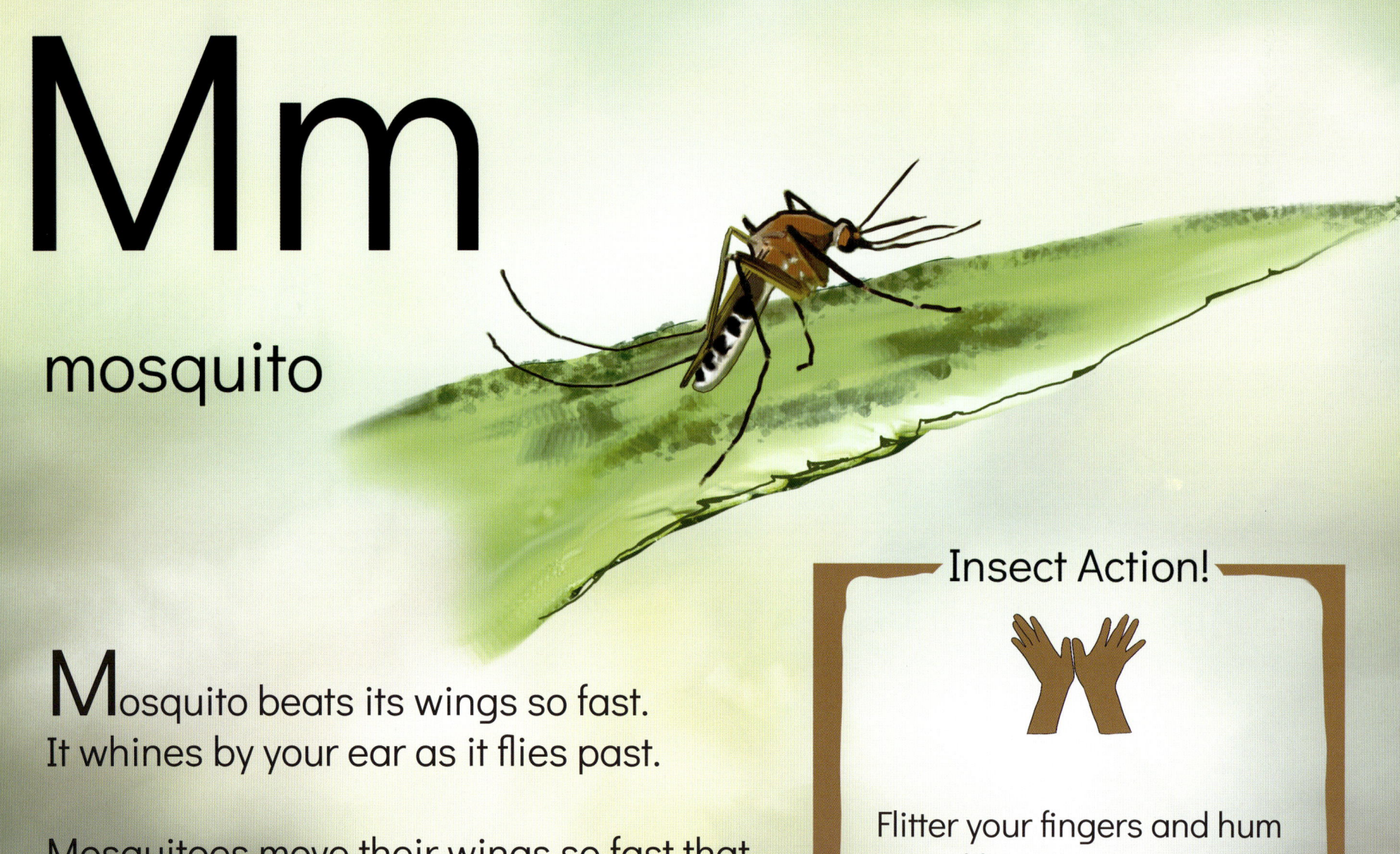

Mosquito beats its wings so fast. It whines by your ear as it flies past.

Mosquitoes move their wings so fast that they make a high-pitched sound. Only the female mosquito bites.

Insect Action!

Flitter your fingers and hum like a mosquito.

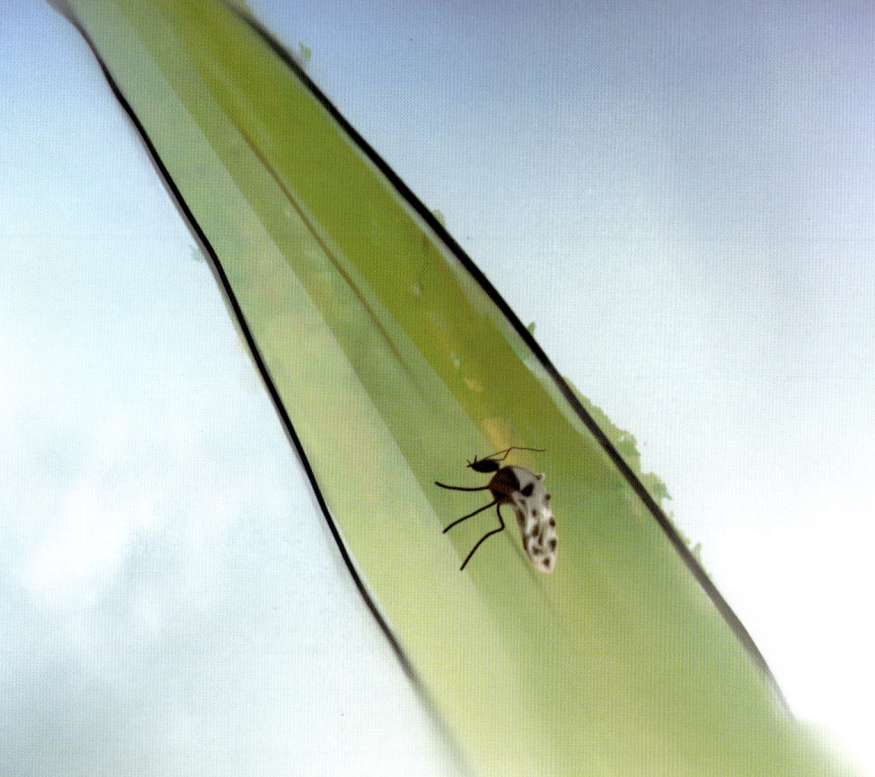

Nn

no-see-um

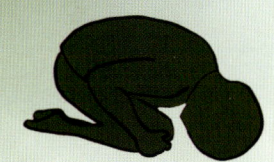
No-see-um, as tiny as can be, may leave a spot that is quite itchy.

No-see-ums are hard to see because of their size. They are pests that may leave an itchy red mark on your skin.

Oo

owl butterfly

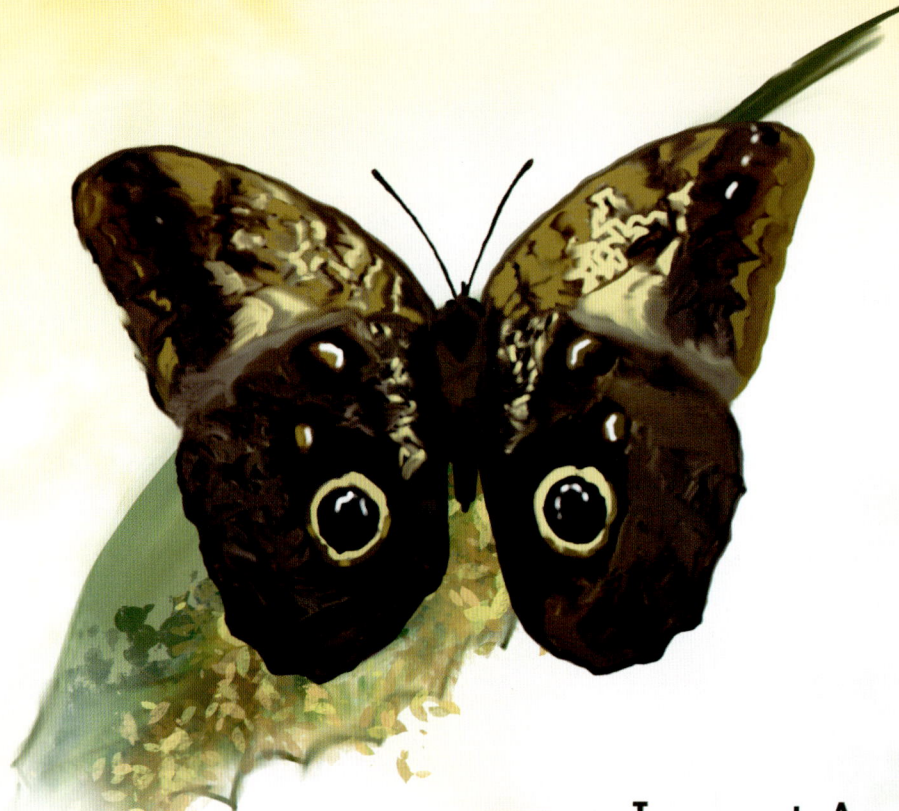

Owl butterfly has spots like eyes. It fools predators with this *disguise*!

Owl butterflies have round spots on their wings that look like an owl's eyes, which frighten away predators. They are active at dawn and dusk.

Insect Action!

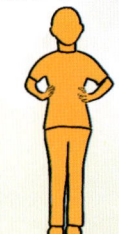

Form circles with each arm at your sides and move your arms back and forth like an owl butterfly.

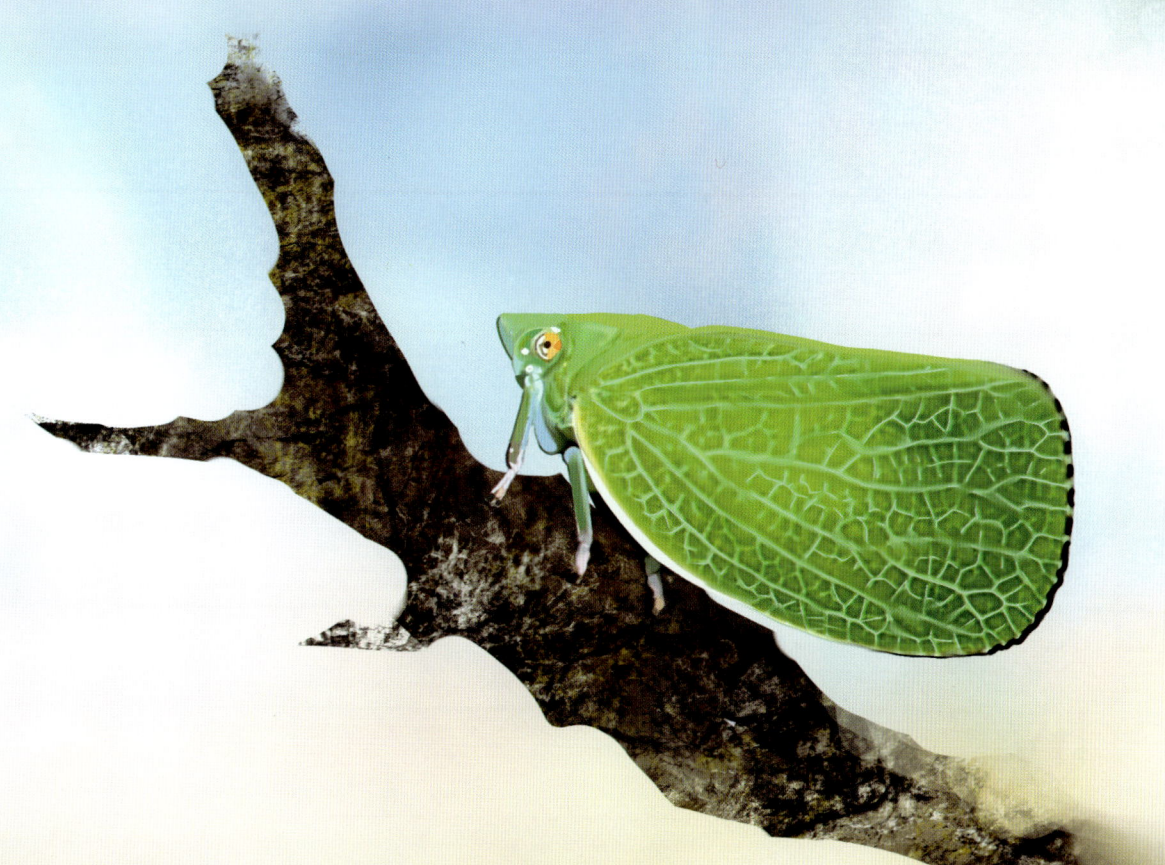

Pp
planthopper

Insect Action!

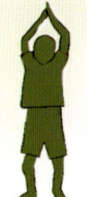 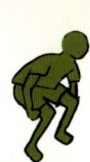 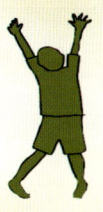

Put your hands together up high and hop like a planthopper.

Planthopper hops from plant to plant. It can walk slow—but run it can't!

Planthoppers look like leaves standing up and use camouflage to hide among leafy plants. They hop very quickly to move about.

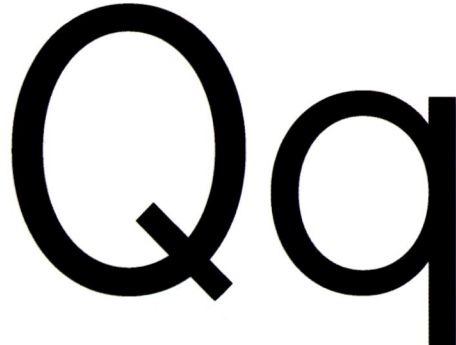

Qq

Queen Alexandra's birdwing butterfly

Queen Alexandra's birdwing, black and blue—
the size of each wing is as big as a toddler's shoe!

Queen Alexandra's birdwing butterflies are the largest butterflies in the world.

Insect Action!

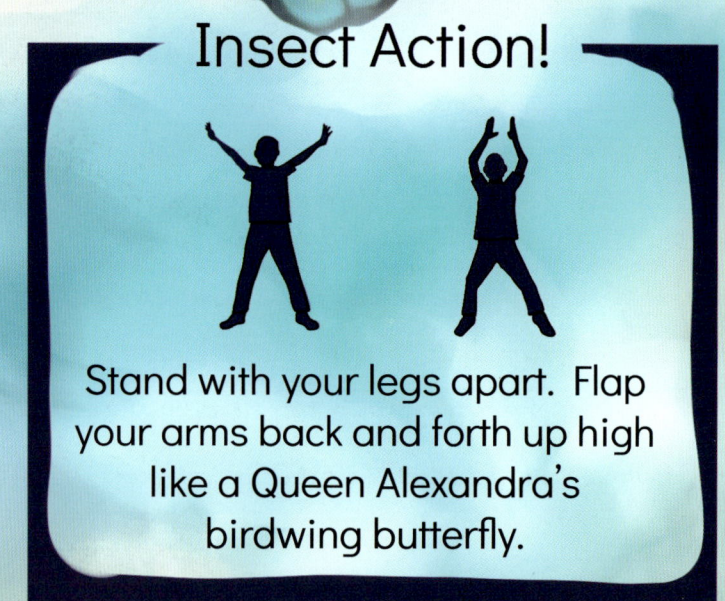

Stand with your legs apart. Flap your arms back and forth up high like a Queen Alexandra's birdwing butterfly.

Rr

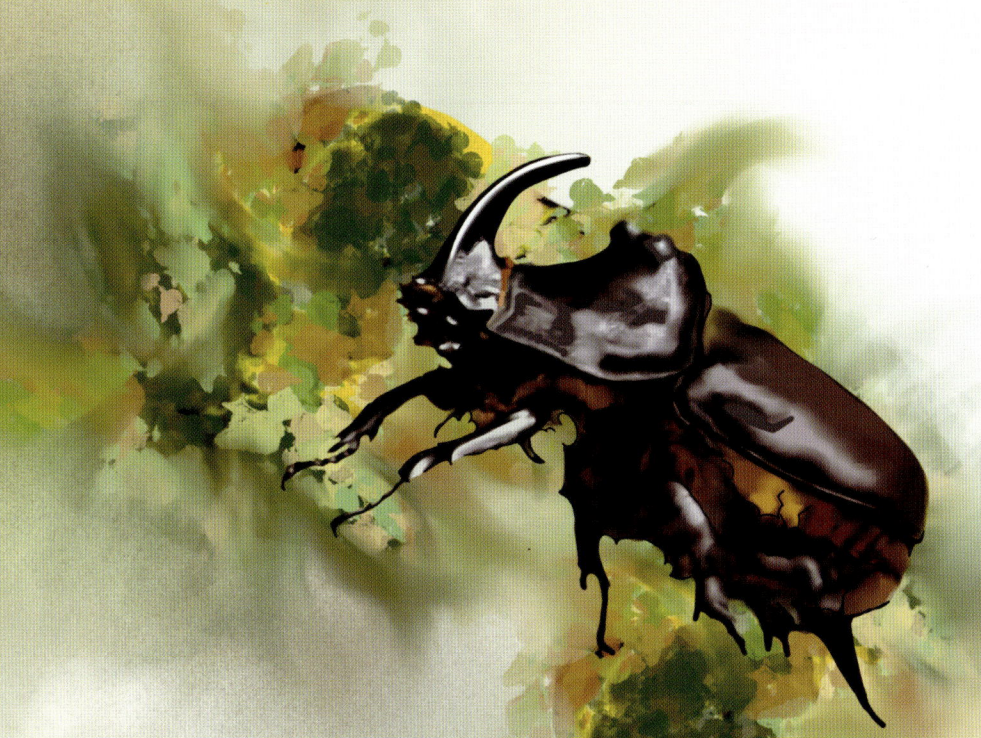

rhinoceros beetle

Insect Action!

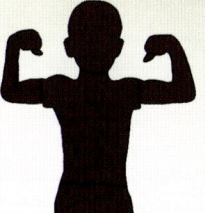

Show your muscles big and strong like a rhinoceros beetle.

Rhinoceros beetle is big and strong. It has one horn that curves quite long.

Rhinoceros beetles look fierce, but they are harmless to people.

Ss

stink bug

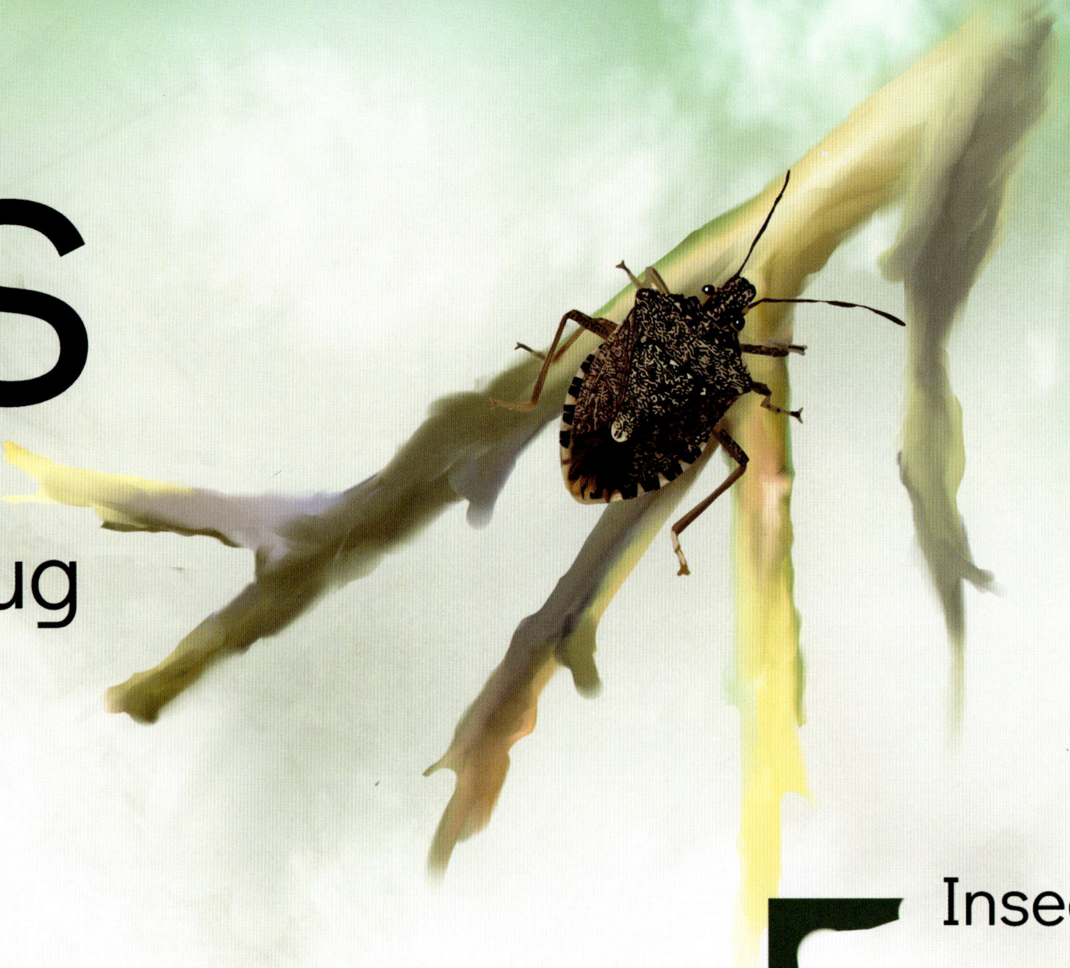

Stink bug really does stink, you know.
Gardeners would rather see it go!

Stink bugs are plant eaters. They may
spray a stinky liquid if they feel
threatened.

Insect Action!

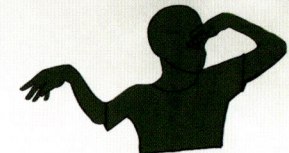

Hold your nose shut and
wave your hand like you
smell a stink bug. Pew!

Tt

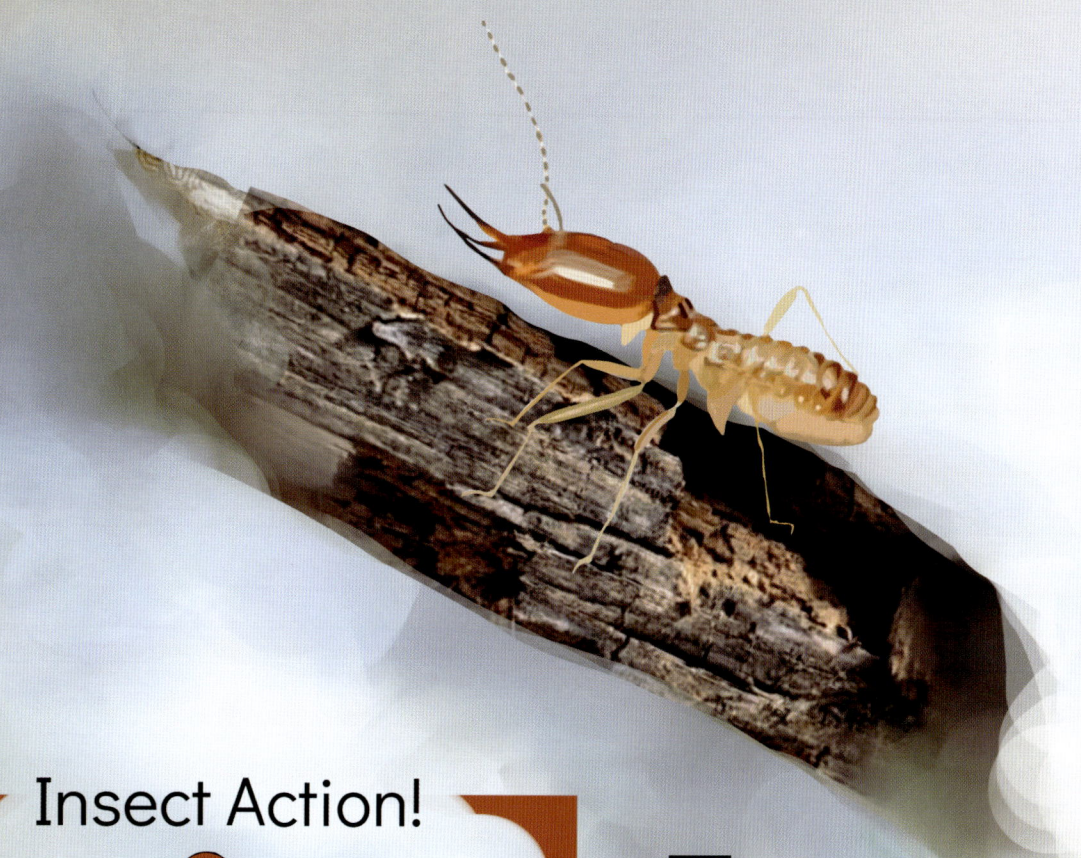

termite

Insect Action!

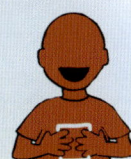

Open and close your mouth to munch like a hungry termite.

Termites munch on leaves and wood. Keeping them out of your house would be good!

Termites are very busy and never sleep. They like to eat plants and wood, and can even damage a house.

Uu

underwing moth

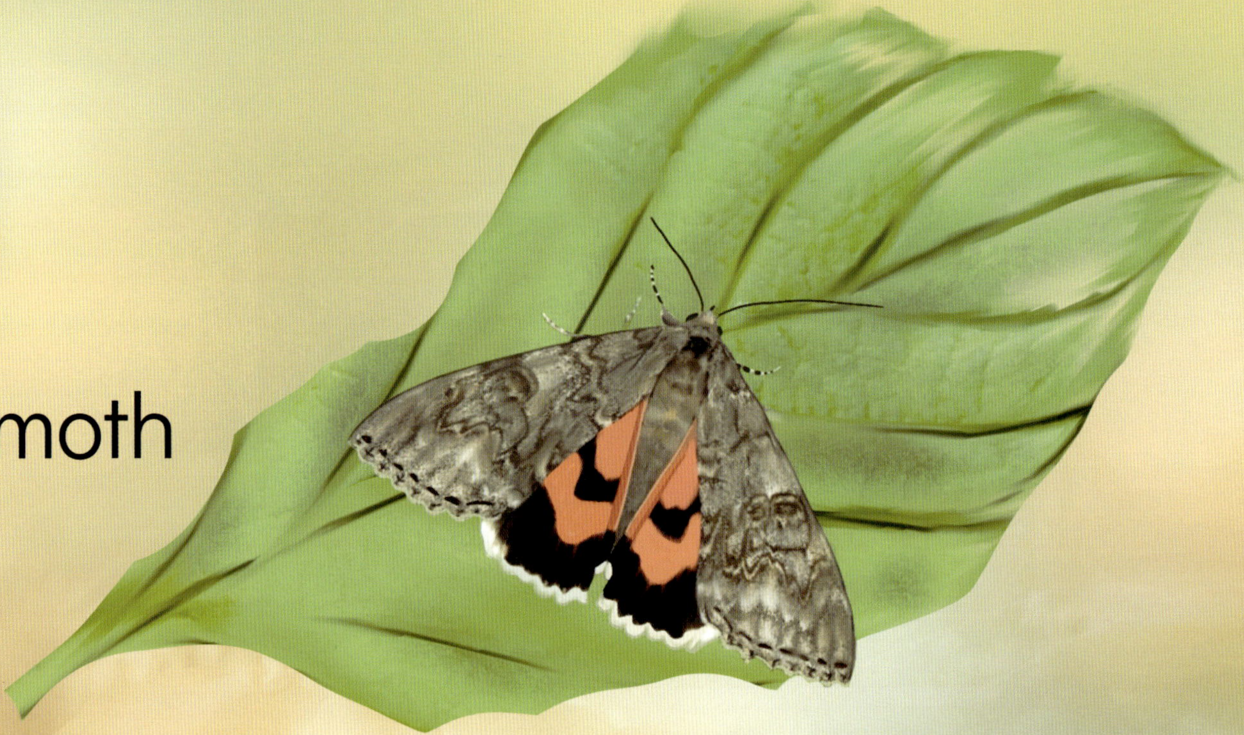

Underwing moth's wings may not all show,
two large on top and two small below.

Underwing moths hide their lower wings
when they rest.

Insect Action!

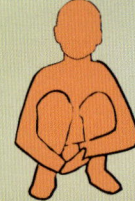

Crouch with your knees bent.
Hide your legs under your
arms like an underwing moth.

Vv

velvet ant

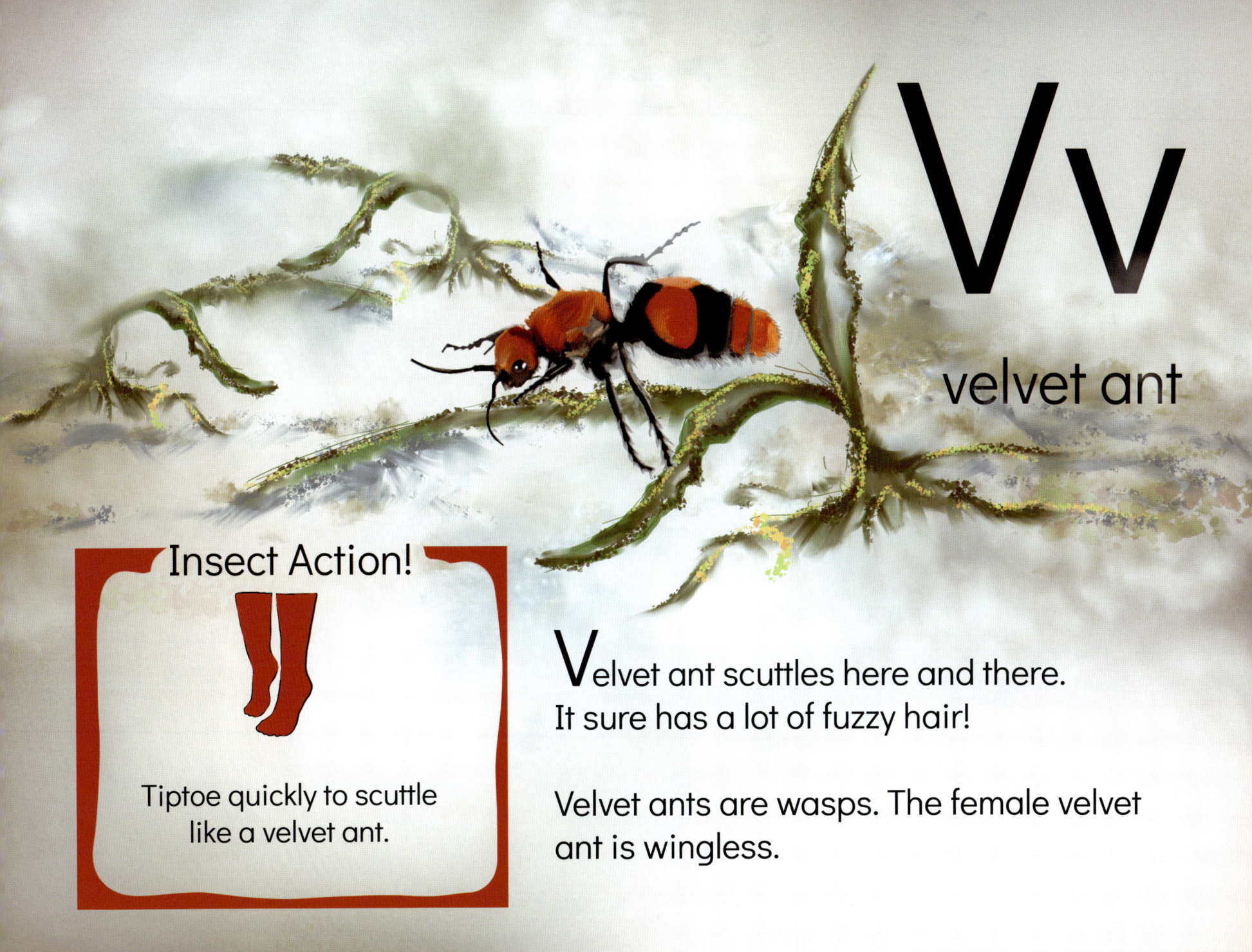

Insect Action!

Tiptoe quickly to scuttle like a velvet ant.

Velvet ant scuttles here and there. It sure has a lot of fuzzy hair!

Velvet ants are wasps. The female velvet ant is wingless.

Ww

walking stick

Walking stick is long and slender.
Among the twigs, it's a great pretender.

Walking sticks look like twigs and may be
hard to spot among other twigs. They walk
very slowly, sometimes swaying back and
forth to resemble a twig moving in the breeze.

Insect Action!

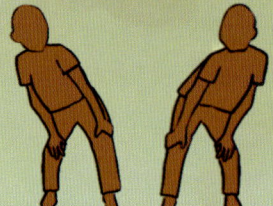

Crouch with your hands on
your knees and sway back
and forth like a walking stick.

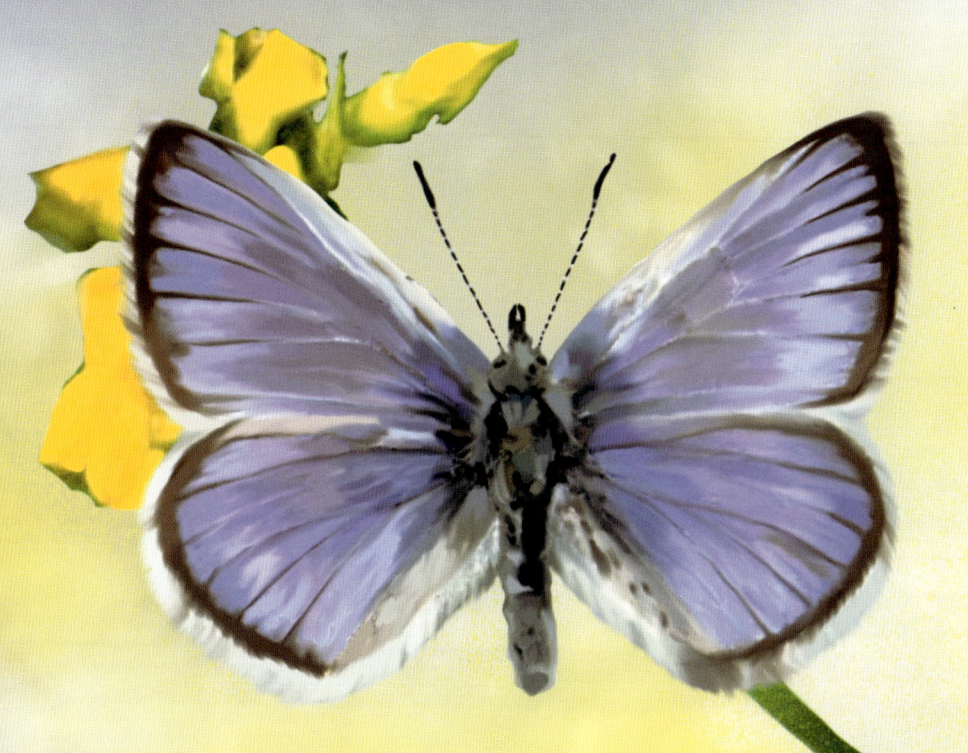

Xx

Xerces blue butterfly

Insect Action!

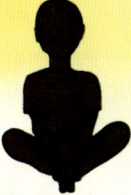

Sit with your feet together and knees out to the sides. Move your legs up and down like a Xerces blue butterfly.

Xerces blue butterfly isn't here today—it's *extinct*, like dinosaurs, sad to say.

Xerces blue butterflies had small, delicate wings. They disappeared after their *habitat* was disturbed.

Yy

yellow jacket

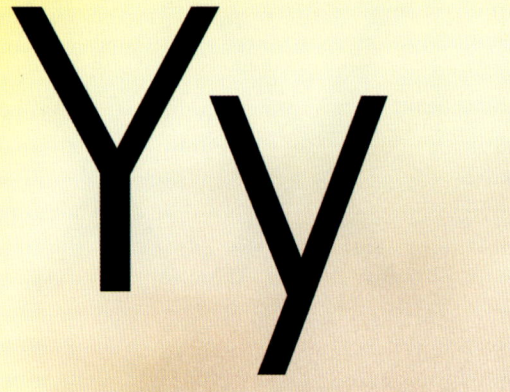

Yellow jacket sniffs for sweets in summer, swooping near your treats—what a bummer!

Yellow jackets are attracted to sweet things. These wasps are common pests at picnics.

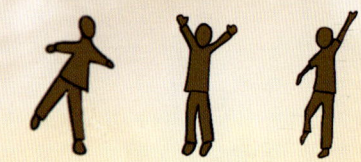

Insect Action!

Swoop back and forth and sniff the air like a yellow jacket.

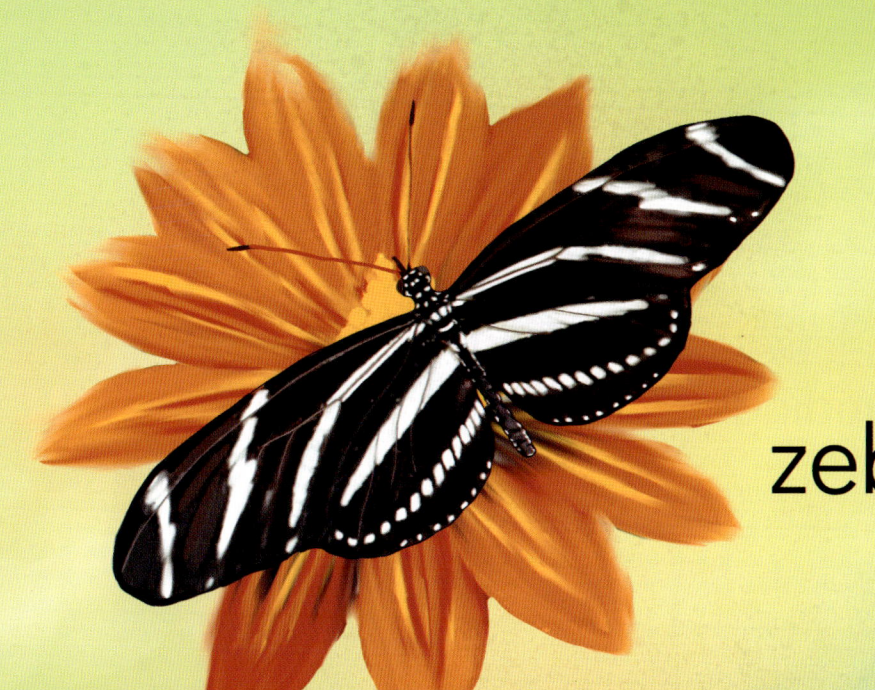

Zz

zebra longwing butterfly

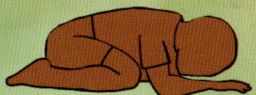
Zebra longwing butterfly moves with grace, and when it sleeps, it shares its space.

Zebra longwing butterflies **roost** at night in groups.

Words to Know

Abdomen: the last section of an insect's body behind its legs

Agility: being able to move around quickly and easily

Camouflage: to blend in with surroundings

Communicate: to share news

Disguise: to look like something else

Extinct: none are living

Habitat: the area where a creature lives naturally

Insects: creatures that have six legs and three body parts

Iridescent: having brilliant colors that change depending on how you look at it

Nocturnal: active at night

Predators: creatures that capture and eat others

Propelling: causing something to get moving

Roost: to settle down for rest or sleep

Activities to Extend Learning

- Make up your own insect movements.

- Find insects where you live.

- Draw a picture of your favorite insect.

- Create an insect using paper, recycled materials, or modeling clay.

- Identify rhyming words in the book.

- Identify nouns, verbs, and adjectives in the book.

- Write a story about an insect.

- Do further research on an insect.

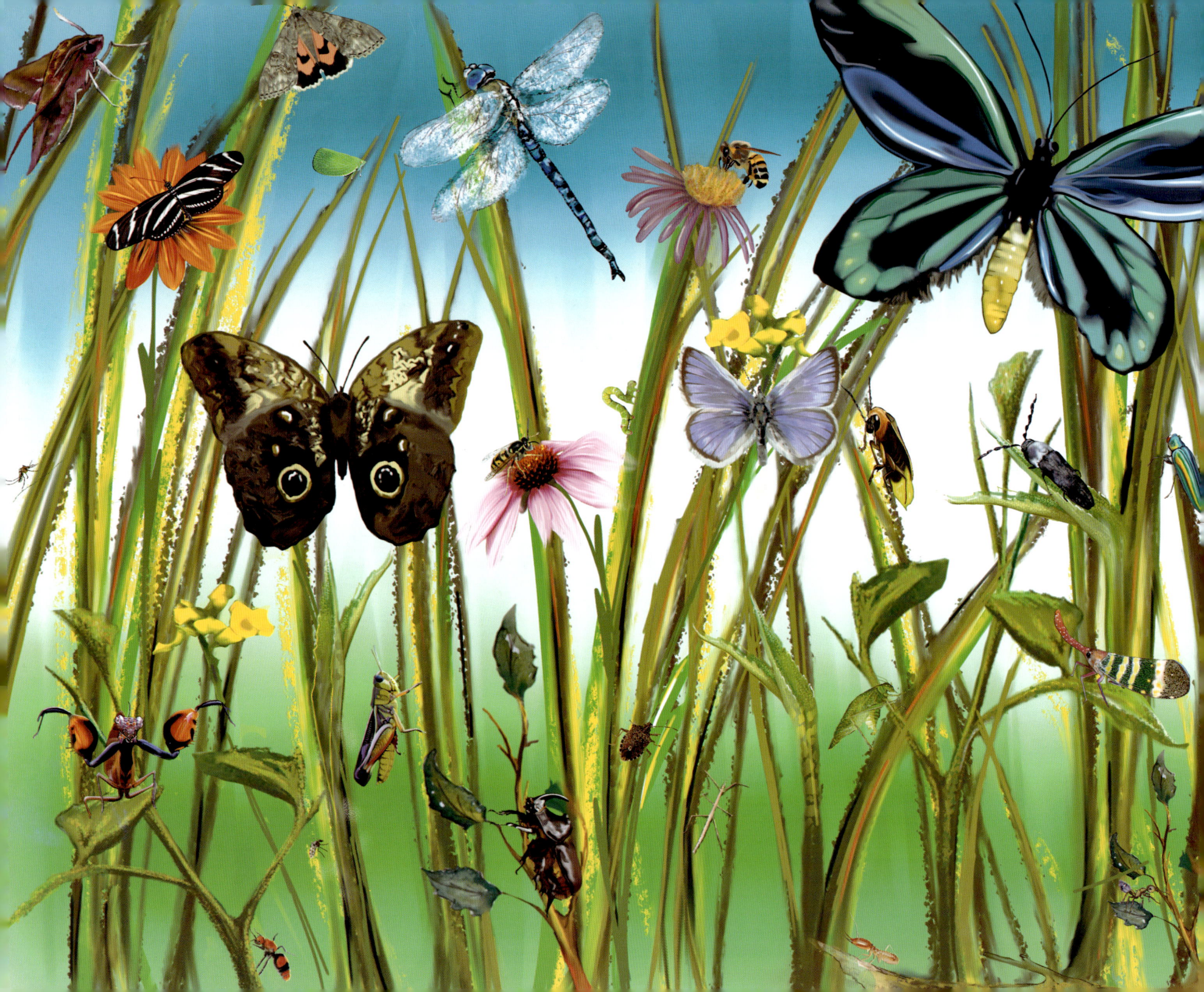